SKIN
PROBLEMS

HERBAL REMEDIES

SKIN PROBLEMS

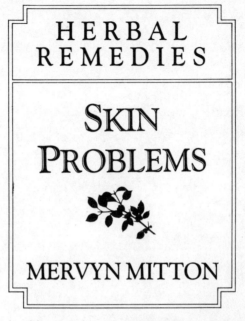

MERVYN MITTON

Edited by David Potterton ND, MRN, MNIMH
*Consultant Medical Herbalist and
Registered Naturopath*

foulsham

LONDON · NEW YORK · TORONTO · SYDNEY

foulsham

Yeovil Road, Slough, Berkshire SL1 4JH

ISBN 0-572-01710-3

Printed by St Edmundsbury Press, Bury St Edmunds, Suffolk.
Phototypeset by Typesetting Solutions, Slough, Berks.

Preface

In the early years of this century most medicines were based on herbs. Indeed, many remedies prescribed by doctors had been used with success down the centuries. Even as late as the 1940s about half of all prescriptions still contained herbal ingredients.

During the sixties and seventies, the medical profession began to discard the older, proven methods of treatment in favour of newer chemical-based drugs. Although pharmaceutical research has produced life-saving drugs, there have also been unfortunate results due to the over-reliance on drug therapy for less serious ailments. We now frequently hear reports of side effects — some of them serious — from many of these relatively untested medicines. A number of drugs have had to be withdrawn from the market.

Within the last few years, however, there has been a dramatic resurgence of interest, both from the medical profession and the public, in alternative and complementary forms of treatment, of which herbal medicine remains the most popular.

The aim of this book is to help signpost your way to the many possibilities for safe home treatment with herbs. However, if any doubts about treatment arise it is advisable to seek professional help from a qualified medical herbalist.

The author, Mr Mitton, was a consulting herbalist at Cathay of Bournemouth, a large retail herbal business established by his parents many years ago.

This revised edition of his book gives relevant information and advice to the seeker of good health who wishes to know more about herbal medicine.

5

Contents

Introduction

There is no doubt that skin ailments are a great source of worry to many sufferers — often out of all proportion to the extent of the affected area.

Several forms of psoriasis are particularly distressing, and can cause great embarrassment, so much so that some patients are prevented from leaving their homes. Since psoriasis often has nervous origins, this additional tension and worry creates a vicious circle which, unfortunately, leads to further inflammation.

Unlike the orthodox medical approach, which is to make a diagnosis and treat the symptoms of the disease, medical herbalists always take a holistic view so that contributing causes are taken into account as well as the presenting symptoms.

The logic of the balanced approach quickly becomes apparent during consultations when it can be seen how one condition can be associated, and indeed, become responsible for others. For example, nervous tension can be responsible for hair loss and loss of condition; stomach ulcers and indigestion; and skin complaints such as psoriasis.

To treat just the symptoms and ignore the original cause, as in the above example of nervous tension, is obviously not going to provide a complete answer, since the problem is likely to reassert itself the next time the sufferer comes under strain.

With herbal treatment it is important to remember that provided it is used correctly there will generally be no side-effects. Herbal medicines are not addictive and do not require ever-increasing dosages to maintain their effect.

The remedies recommended in this book are all based on the known properties of individual herbs. In most cases they can be prepared and taken at home which is important since experience shows that many people who suffer disorders prefer to try to control the problem themselves before seeking professional help.

This does not imply that where a serious medical condition exists it should be treated at home from the advice given in this book. In such a case the best advice is always to seek the opinion of a physician or qualified medical herbalist. However, where the pattern of the problem matches examples given, or where the advice is applicable, herbal treatment could well provide the answer.

Chapter 1

Identifying your illness

It is likely that most people suffering from psoriasis or other skin disorders will have already sought medical advice and have had a correct diagnosis made. However, sometimes complications arise, or the condition is not thought serious enough to worry the doctor, and it is for this reason that a description of the various illnesses and their symptoms is given.

Many readers will be dedicated already to the use of natural medicines; others may have tried alternative treatments without success. The most important thing is to ensure that you have correctly identified your condition before commencing the treatments outlined here as a misdiagnosis could lead to a deterioration in your health.

Second, remember that herbal treatment is relatively slow-acting and generally relies on a gradual build-up in the system. This makes it particularly suitable for long-term skin complaints since herbs are usually without side-effects, not addictive and are compatible with one another.

ACNE

This is a chronic skin disease due to a disorder of the sebaceous glands of the face, chest and shoulders. It often breaks out at puberty, and clears by the early twenties.

9

The eruptions of acne can take several forms, from pustules to hard lumps. In treating acne, care must be taken to remove surface bacteria and allow the pustules to heal naturally. Too much interference can result in scarring. Diet is important and constipation should be treated.

Herbal treatment: try the *Herb Mixture for Skin Eruptions* and for external use *A Herbal Antiseptic Lotion*. A consultation with a qualified medical herbalist would be very worthwhile.

ATHLETE'S FOOT

A common problem for those accustomed to walking barefoot in areas of heavy public use such as swimming pools. This is a fungal infection and daily treatment should include regular washing, use of a foot powder between the toes and in socks and shoes. Regular use of the herb poultice (details in Chapter 4) could prove helpful.

BOILS

Usually originating at the base of hairs, these are most common at the back of the neck and on the front part of arms and legs. Generally, they are a sign of being tired and run down and, if they occur regularly, further medical advice should be sought.

A helpful herb mixture for boils is given in Chapter 4.

BRUISES

Usually as the result of a knock, blood escapes into the surrounding skin tissue, leading to the darkened blue/black appearance.

A cold compress can be helpful and also regular

applications of the *Herbal Lotion for Cuts, Bruises and Burns* (see Chapter 4).

DERMATITIS

This is an inflammation of the skin, usually caused by an allergy or by an external irritant — oil, chemicals and grease are typical examples. Dermatitis is not infectious.

Treatment must include avoidance, or protection from, the substance causing the problem. Regular application of the *Herb Mixture for Dermatitis* (see Chapter 4) can be helpful.

ECZEMA

The two main ways of identifying eczema are irritations and blistering of the skin. There are several varieties of this condition, including a hereditary type. Eczema does not always respond well to treatment, but the herbal formula will be found to be of benefit and for external use, the *Herb Mixture for Dermatitis* (see Chapter 4). Sufferers are advised to see a qualified medical herbalist.

LEG ULCERS

Varicose eczema is not to be confused with the above, but is a surface inflammation of the lower part of the leg. It can be a sign of a varicose ulcer forming and is common among older women who have had a family. Excessive standing and sitting should be avoided. The general circulation needs to be improved. Of other forms of ulcers, callous ulcers are the most common, with a hard, thick edge.

Ulcers can occur in various parts of the body but, understandably, leg ulcers cause much anguish. Herbal treatment has proved effective by improving the blood circulation as well as treating the actual ulcer. Rest, elevation of the affected leg and correct bandaging is also most important.

Formulae for a herbal poultice and a simple ointment are given in Chapter 4. Diagnosis is important, and it would be helpful to consult a medical herbalist.

PRURITUS ANI/VULVAE

This is skin irritation affecting the anal and vaginal area. Candida may be one cause of the condition. Specific herb treatments are included in Chapter 4.

PSORIASIS

This skin disease can be hereditary. But it is usually associated with nervous tension, since a severe nervous or emotional shock will often precipitate it. It will often break out again after lying dormant, or increase in intensity when the patient comes under increased stress.

Other contributory causes can be rheumatism and gout.

There are several forms of psoriasis ranging from reddening and scaling of the skin to thick encrustations. Treatment could include the *Herb Mixture for Psoriasis*, *Herbal Nerve Mixture* and *Herb Mixture for Skin Eruptions* (see Chapter 4). The surface area should be kept free of bacteria with a medicated soap.

RINGWORM

This is a contagious fungal infection usually affecting the scalps of children. Borage, applied as an infusion, can prove helpful.

SKIN ERUPTIONS

This heading covers problems such as itching, rashes and outbreaks of spots which cannot readily be covered by any of the other specific illnesses. If frequent, diet and possible contributory causes should be looked at. Application of the *Herbal Antiseptic Lotion* will usually help. Also take the *Herb Mixture for Skin Eruptions* internally (see Chapter 4).

WARTS

These are small lumps of hard matter growing from the skin surface. They are due to a viral infection and are very common. Sometimes they occur in clusters. The most common place for warts is on the hands, but there are other types which can grow on the face, body, feet and genitals and even internally. When dealing with warts, the formula given in Chapter 4 will be of help, but instructions should be followed closely and only one or two dealt with at a time. Warts growing in sensitive places, i.e. on the face or around genitals should be dealt with by a qualified medical herbalist or physician.

Chapter 2

Some commonly used drugs

This chapter outlines some of the drugs prescribed by doctors for the treatment of various skin diseases, together with some of the side effects and adverse reactions associated with them. Some of the drugs listed in the first edition of this book have been withdrawn, or reformulated, or have been replaced by more modern preparations.

The information has not been given to alarm anyone who may be using any of these drugs, but to make them aware of their possible effects. However, it should be emphasised that people react differently to drugs and that not everyone will, necessarily, suffer side effects.

I believe that many doctors fail to explain fully to their patients the side effects that can be expected from a particular drug, or course of treatment, and that this may cause great distress. This is often due to a failure to communicate since pharmaceutical companies usually advise doctors of the side effects reported during the clinical trials of their medicines.

While there are a number of drugs used for dermatological conditions which are not listed here, and which are deemed to have fewer side effects, it should be remembered that all chemical-based drugs are expected to produce side effects.

There is often more than one proprietary brand of a drug, particularly where the patent for the original drug has expired. Brand names are given in brackets.

AMPHOTERICIN
(Fungilin)
(Fungizone)

Indications: Fungal infections.

Possible side effects: Gastrointestinal upset.

BACITRACIN

Indications: Bacterial infections of the skin.

Possible side effects: Used mainly in combination with other drugs and may give rise to allergic reactions.

CLOBETASONE BUTYRATE
(Eumovate)

Indications: Eczema, seborrhoeic dermatitis and other skin disorders responsive to steroid treatment.

Possible side effects: A moderately potent steroid which may have adverse effects on the skin and blood capillaries if overused.

DITHRANOL
(Anthranol)

Indications: Chronic psoriasis.

Possible side effects: Irritation and burning of the skin. Hypersensitivity reactions.

GRISEOFULVIN
(Fulcin)
(Grisovin)

Indications: Internal treatment for fungal infections of scalp, nail and skin when local applications have failed.

Possible side effects: Headache, drowsiness, stomach upsets, skin rashes, sensitivity of the skin to light.

ITRACONAZOLE
(Sporonox)

Indications: Pityriasis versicolor, fungal skin conditions.

Possible side effects: Indigestion, nausea, headache, painful abdomen. May interact with antacids and ulcer drugs.

METHOTREXATE
(Maxtrex)

Indications: Severe psoriasis which does not respond to other treatments.

Possible side effects: Gastrointestinal and liver disturbance, rashes. May also interfere with bone marrow function.

RESORCINAL

Indications: Used in ointments to cause peeling of the skin in acne vulgaris.

Possible side effects: Skin irritation. Overuse may interfere with thyroid function.

TERBINAFINE
(Lamisil)

Indications: Fungal infections of the skin requiring internal treatment.

Possible side effects: Gastrointestinal upset, allergic skin reactions, nausea.

TRIAMCINOLONE ACETONIDE
(Adcortyl)
(Ledercort)

Indications: Inflammatory skin conditions, dermatitis, psoriasis, insect bites, sunburn.

Possible side effects: A potent steroid in a cream or ointment base which may have adverse effects on the skin and blood capillaries if overused.

Chapter 3

Some problems which trouble sufferers

Skin ailments, particularly if they are visible and cannot be easily covered by clothing, can cause great embarrassment and loss of confidence in the sufferer. For someone unlucky enough to have a facial rash, acne or psoriasis on the hands or knees, it can take great courage to appear in public and, of course, it is not unusual for additional problems of nervous tension quickly to present themselves. With the balanced approach of herbal medicine, which treats not only the effect but also seeks to find the original cause and treat this as well, a good success rate can be achieved.

The success of this approach has been amply demonstrated to me on numerous occasions. I have seen teenagers coming into our shops to purchase our recommendations for acne. Obviously, they have already bought various proprietary brands of skin creams, but since these treat only the surface problem and do not attempt to deal with the internal causes, their effects rarely last for long. Therefore, the message spreads by word of mouth that a combination of the two treatments, i.e. internal and external, can be effective and they come in for help. For a young man in his mid-teens to seek out and make such a purchase, shows just how much of a mental problem acne can be for him.

Psoriasis is a good example of a problem where both the

cause and the effect must be treated. In my experience it can often be brought on by a severe emotional shock and, even when various types of treatment clear it, there is always the possibility that renewed tension will cause it to recur. Treatment for psoriasis, therefore, particularly when the nervous origin can be clearly established, must include something safe to calm the nervous system, in addition to treating the skin surface. There are, of course, alternative causes for psoriasis, including heredity and internal disturbance. In the case of the latter, herbal treatment can also be given.

Although herbal medicine is becoming more widely accepted today, many people still believe that only chemical drugs can be effective. But drugs, particularly for skin diseases, are prone to cause side effects. In many cases drugs have been withdrawn.

I am reminded of a particular example which shows the effectiveness of traditional herbal medication against the modern chemical 'wonder' drugs. A woman living on the South Coast came to me for help after suffering for over five years from a fungal-type infection on her chin. This had resulted in thickened patches of red skin and in a white sticky matter being expelled through the pores.

She had received treatment both at local hospitals and from skin specialists, none of whom had identified the problem and, on at least two occasions, the side effects of the drugs prescribed had caused her very serious problems. When she came to see me, there had been an increase in the activity of the affected area which was spreading and expelling more matter than usual.

After consideration, I recommended a poultice of Marshmallow combined with Slippery Elm to be placed, twice daily, over the affected area. The poultice was to be as warm as possible and left on for at least twenty minutes. As a skin lotion, I recommended an infusion of Fumitory and Burdock Root. After just four days a root system appeared to be coming out through the pores, something which had never happened during the previous five years of treatment and, within two to three weeks, a large percentage of the area was clearing up.

The properties of all of these herbal remedies have been known for hundreds of years, but in the correct combination they were able to quickly commence healing, something that modern drugs had been unable to touch. Proof indeed that traditional herbal medicine used in the right way, and for the right illnesses, is still effective.

Chapter 4

Herbal treatments and formulae

The following formulae are all suitable to make up as directed, using quantities shown as percentages of the whole.

Ingredients should be available from medical herbalists, herbal retailers and many health food shops — if any difficulty is experienced consult the list of addresses at the back of the book.

INFORMATION ON THE PREPARATION OF HERBS

DECOCTIONS
The herbs are cut, ground up or bruised and covered with cold fresh water. This mixture is then boiled for up to half an hour, allowed to cool and then strained through a fine mesh. Allow 28 grams of the herbs to 568 ml of water (1 oz to 1 pint). This method is normally used when the herb is unsuitable to make as an infusion. The usual dose is approximately one small wineglassful three times daily.

INFUSIONS
Teas or tisanes are made by the process of infusion. Prepare the herbs to be used and quickly pour boiling water on them. Allow the mixture to stand for about half an hour, stirring frequently, and when ready, strain off the liquid. Allow 28 grams to 568 ml of water (1 oz to 1 pint).

The usual dose is approximately one small teacup or wineglassful three times daily. Usually one after each main meal.

SOLID EXTRACTS
Start with a strong infusion of the herbs required and evaporate over low heat until a heavy consistency is obtained.

TINCTURES
This process is used for herbs and drugs which become useless when heated, or for those herbs which are not amenable to treatment by water. Tinctures are made commercially with pure alcohol. Use 28 to 56 grams to 568 ml (1 or 2 oz to 1 pint). The dose varies according to the strength of the main ingredient. For home use tinctures can be made with brandy, but this is rather an expensive process.

POWDER
Some herbs may be easily prepared as a powder by grating or applying pressure to them. More usually, powder will be a form in which the herb can be purchased. Depending on its intended use, a powdered herb may be used externally as a poultice or, if suitable, can be taken internally by sprinkling in food, mixing it with a fluid or as an electuary by mixing the appropriate amount with an equal amount of honey. For the dose, start with a small amount (¼ tsp or less) 2 or 3 times daily and gradually increase until the desired benefits are obtained.

SOME SIMPLE FORMULAE TO MAKE AT HOME

A HERB MIXTURE FOR PSORIASIS
Mountain Grape	1 part
Burdock Root	1 part

Yellow Dock Root	1 part
Red Clover Flowers	1 part
Sarsaparilla	1 part

Make up as an infusion.

A HERB MIXTURE FOR ECZEMA

Fumitory	1 part
Clivers	1 part
Burdock Root	1 part
Yellow Dock Root	1 part
Nettle	1 part

Make up as an infusion.

A HERB MIXTURE FOR DERMATITIS

| Irish Moss | 1 part |
| Golden Seal | 1 part |

Make up as a decoction. *External application only.*

A HERB MIXTURE FOR BOILS

Echinacea	1 part
Blue Flag	1 part
Pulsatilla	1 part
Wild Indigo	1 part

Make up as a decoction.

A HERB MIXTURE FOR ATHLETE'S FOOT

| Comfrey Leaf | 1 part |
| Linseed | 1 part |

Make up as a poultice and apply warm to affected area.

A HERB MIXTURE FOR PRURITIS VULVAE

Lady's Mantle

Make up as an infusion. Apply *externally* as a warm douche.

A HERB MIXTURE FOR PRURITIS ANI

Golden Seal	1 part
Witch Hazel Leaf	1 part
Passiflora	1 part

Make up as an infusion. Apply *externally* to affected areas.

A HERB MIXTURE FOR SKIN ERUPTIONS

Wild Indigo	1 part
Echinacea	1 part
Pulsatilla	1 part

Make up as a decoction.

A HERB MIXTURE FOR WARTS

Greater Celandine	1 part
Thuja	1 part

For external use only. Bruise 25 g (1 oz) of mixed herbs by pounding with a heavy instrument. Steep in 25 g (1 oz) alcohol (gin or vodka is suitable for this purpose) for 48 hours. Strain the liquid, and bottle. Cut a plaster to fit around the wart to be treated and dab the liquid on to the wart several times daily. Avoid delicate areas and treat only one or two warts at a time. (See Chapter 1.)

HERB POULTICE FOR LEG ULCERS

Slippery Elm Bark	1 part
Marshmallow Root	1 part
Comfrey Root	1 part

Boil up the herbs together. When they are sufficiently cool, apply externally as a poultice to the ulcer. Bind lightly or hold in position for one to two hours.

A SIMPLE OINTMENT FOR LEG ULCERS

Wild Indigo Root	1 part
Petroleum Jelly BP	8 parts

(*Vaseline* is a branded form of Petroleum Jelly.)

Make a decoction of Wild Indigo Root. Strain. Add the liquid to the petroleum jelly in the proportions shown. Bring to the boil and ensure the two combine. Skim the top and pour into a clean jar when cool. Allow to set and put on an airtight cap.

Apply the ointment to clean lint and gently lay over the ulcer. Hold in position with a loose bandage. Change dressing every day.

Note: Be careful when changing the dressing not to break the 'healing ring' of the ulcer, this is on the outside edge and gradually closes the ulcer towards the middle.

A HERBAL ANTISEPTIC LOTION

Marigold	1 part
Golden Seal	1 part
Pulsatilla	1 part

Make up as an infusion. Strain thoroughly. Apply as required to the affected area.

A HERBAL LOTION FOR CUTS AND BRUISES

Marigold	1 part
Irish Moss	1 part
Slippery Elm Bark	1 part

Make up as a decoction. Strain thoroughly. Apply as required.

A HERB FOR THE TREATMENT OF RINGWORM
Borage

Make up as an infusion. *External use only.* Apply to the affected area several times daily.

A HERBAL NERVE MIXTURE FOR USE IN CASES OF PSORIASIS

Motherwort	1 part
Hops	1 part
Vervain	1 part
Lime Flowers	1 part
Scullcap	1 part

Make up as an infusion.

Chapter 5

Some recommended herbs

This section of the book lists in alphabetical order some of the herbs which can be used in the treatment of conditions mentioned earlier, together with other herbs of a generally beneficial nature.

A list of herbal suppliers is given at the end of the section. A few herbal medicines may be available only on prescription from a medical herbalist.

Mitton's Practical Modern Herbal, published by Foulsham, is recommended for a more complete list of medical herbs and their uses, together with much useful and practical information.

Acacia Gum
ACACIA SENEGAL

Also known as	Gum Arabic.
Found wild	North Africa.
Appearance	Round tears obtained from spring shrub. Cuts are made in the bark and the gum exudes and coagulates.
Part used	Coagulated gum.
Therapeutic uses	An excellent demulcent — often used to relieve catarrh and chest complaints.
Prepared as	Mucilage by combining hot water with the gum.

29

Adder's Tongue (American)
ERYTHRONIUM AMERICANUM

Also known as	Snake's Tongue.
Found wild	North America.
Appearance	Small bulbous plant with only two leaves and bright yellow lily-like flowers.
Part used	Leaves.
Therapeutic uses	Generally as a poultice for ulcers and skin troubles.
Prepared as	Poultice.

Agar-Agar
GELIDIUM AMANSII

Also known as	Japanese Isinglass.
Found wild	Japan.
Appearance	Several different seaweeds are made into thin strips of about 30 cm/12 inches long.
Part used	Translucent strips.
Therapeutic uses	Excellent for relief of stubborn constipation.
Prepared as	Powder.

Agrimony
AGRIMONIA EUPATORIA

Also known as	Sticklewort.
Found wild	Throughout northern Europe.

Appearance	A strong growing herb with green/grey leaves covered with soft hairs. Flowers are small and yellow on long slender spikes.
Part used	Herb.
Therapeutic uses	Dried leaves when infused make an astringent useful for skin eruptions, pimples and blotches. Also as a tonic and diuretic. Used in cases of simple diarrhoea.
Prepared as	Infusion.

Alder (English)
ALNUS GLUTINOSA

Found wild	England, Europe and North Africa.
Appearance	A small tree of distinctive appearance.
Parts used	Bark and leaves.
Therapeutic uses	The bark is used as a cathartic and the leaves to treat inflammatory conditions.
Prepared as	Decoction and poultice.

Aloes
ALOE VERA

| **Also known as** | Cape Aloes. |

Found wild	Southern Africa and West Indies.
Appearance	Fleshy, prickly succulent plant of medium height. Evergreen.
Part used	Sap dried as powder.
Therapeutic uses	Used as a purgative and expellent of intestinal worms. Also used to promote the menses.
Prepared as	Decoction.

Alstonia Bark
ALSTONIA CONSTRICTA

Also known as	Fever Bark or Australia Quinine.
Found wild	Australia.
Appearance	Thick chocolate-coloured spongy bark from a moderate size tree.
Part used	Bark.
Therapeutic uses	To prevent recurring bouts of malaria and for quick relief of most forms of rheumatism.
Prepared as	Decoction.

Amaranth
AMARANTHUS HYPOCHONDRIACUS

Also known as	Love Lies Bleeding.
Found wild	UK and Europe.
Appearance	A common garden plant with crimson flowers.
Part used	Herb.

Therapeutic uses	Treatment of diarrhoea and menorrhagia and as an astringent. Helpful in all cases of looseness of the bowel. Use externally as a wash for skin ulcers and sore patches.
Prepared as	Decoction.

Ammoniacum
DOREMA AMMONIACUM

Also known as	Gum Ammoniacum.
Found wild	Turkey and Iran.
Appearance	Small, rounded lumps, pale yellow in colour and browning with age.
Part used	Gum resin.
Therapeutic uses	For respiratory troubles; relief of catarrh, asthma and bronchitis.
Prepared as	Powder.

Angelica
ANGELICA ARCHANGELICA

Found wild	Europe, Asia.
Appearance	Plant growing from four to six feet high.
Parts used	Root, seeds and herb.
Therapeutic uses	For rheumatic diseases, catarrh, asthma. A stimulant and diaphoretic.
Prepared as	Infusion or decoction.

Arrach
CHENOPODIUM OLIDUM

Also known as	Goat's Arrach.
Found wild	Throughout Europe.
Appearance	A small inconspicuous herb having an unpleasant odour.
Part used	Herb.
Therapeutic uses	As an emmenagogue to bring on menstruation. Also an effective nervine.
Prepared as	Infusion.

Avens
GEUM URBANUM

Also known as	Colewort.
Found wild	Throughout Europe.
Appearance	Low-growing herb with yellow flowers.
Parts used	Herb and root.
Therapeutic uses	To stay bleeding and as a reliable tonic, particularly for women. Also used for treating leucorrhea.
Prepared as	Decoction.

Balm
MELISSA OFFICINALIS

Also known as	Lemon Balm and Sweet Balm.
Found wild	Throughout Europe.

Appearance	A plant up to one metre high, with a lemon odour.
Part used	Leaves.
Therapeutic uses	Most effective for the relief of flatulence and indigestion and induces copious perspiration. Can also be made up into a most pleasant and cooling tea.
Prepared as	Infusion.

Balm of Gilead
POPULUS CANDICANS

Also known as	Several other plants are known as Balm of Gilead.
Found wild	United States and Arabia.
Appearance	Strong gnarled shrub with feathery foliage.
Part used	Buds.
Therapeutic uses	Highly regarded tonic and diuretic. Excellent for chest troubles and rheumatic ailments.
Prepared as	Decoction or tincture.

Balmony
CHELONE GLABRA

Also known as	Turtle Head and Snake Herb.
Found wild	North America.
Appearance	Low sturdy bush with oval dark leaves and white or pink flowers.

Balm of Gilead
POPULUS CANDICANS

Several other plants are known as Balm of Gilead.

Found wild   United States and Arabia.

Appearance   Strong gnarled shrub with feathery foliage.

Part used   Buds.

Therapeutic uses Highly regarded as a tonic and diuretic. Excellent for chest troubles and rheumatic ailments.

Prepared as   Decoction or tincture. An ointment is used for skin diseases.

Balmony
CHELONE GLABRA

Also known as   Turtle Head or Snake Herb.

Found wild   United States and Canada.

Appearance   Low, sturdy bush with oval dark leaves and white or pink flowers.

Part used   Leaves.

Therapeutic uses Regarded as one of the best remedies for liver diseases. It is also antibilious, anthelmintic and a tonic.

Prepared as   Infusion.

Basil
OCIMUM BASILICUM

Also known as   Sweet Basil.

Found wild	Northern Europe.
Appearance	A small plant with a multitude of white and pink flowers. Leaves have a strong clover scent.
Part used	Leaves.
Therapeutic uses	Formerly widely used as a carminative and for culinary purposes.
Prepared as	Infusion.

Bayberry
MYRICA CERIFERA

Also known as	Waxberry, Candleberry.
Found wild	Europe and North America.
Appearance	A medium-growing shrub with a profusion of large white berries.
Part used	Bark.
Therapeutic uses	A strong stimulant. A warming and effective deobstruent and cleanser. Also as a poultice for ulcers.
Prepared as	Infusion.

Bearsfoot (American)
POLYMNIA UVEDALIA

| **Also known as** | Yellow Leaf Cup. |
| **Found wild** | North America. |

Appearance	Low-growing herb chiefly found in ditches and damp places.
Part used	Root.
Therapeutic uses	As a treatment for incontinence and as a gargle for sore throats.
Prepared as	Decoction.

Black Root
LEPTANDRA VIRGINICA

Also known as	Culver's Root.
Found wild	United States.
Appearance	A low-growing herb.
Part used	Rhizome.
Therapeutic uses	A blood purifying mixture. Also as a cathartic, diaphoretic and a liver stimulant.
Prepared as	Decoction.

Bladderwrack
FUCUS VESICULOSUS

Also known as	Seawrack and Kelpware.
Found wild	Around the coasts of Britain.
Appearance	A large trailing seaweed, dark green in colour.
Part used	Dried plant.
Therapeutic uses	Acts on thyroid. Tones up the system and clears the kidneys.
Prepared as	Decoction.

Blue Flag
IRIS VERSICOLOR

Also known as	Flag Lily and Water Flag.
Where found	Extensively planted in gardens throughout Britain.
Appearance	A beautiful plant with arching strap-like leaves and blue, white, yellow or multi-coloured flowers.
Part used	Rhizome.
Therapeutic uses	Principally as a blood purifier, also an alterative, diuretic and cathartic.
Prepared as	Decoction or powder.

Boldo
PEUMUS BOLDUS

Also known as	Boldu.
Found wild	Chile.
Appearance	Medium-sized shrub with dark oval leaves and a strong lemon smell.
Part used	Leaves.
Therapeutic uses	As a liver stimulant. It also has antiseptic properties and is of value to sufferers of catarrh of the bladder.
Prepared as	Decoction.

Found wild	United States.
Appearance	A low-growing herb.
Part used	Rhizome.
Therapeutic uses	A blood purifying mixture. Also used as a cathartic, diaphoretic and a liver stimulant.
Prepared as	Decoction.

Bladderwrack
FUCUS VESICULOSUS

Also known as	Seawrack or Kelpware.
Found wild	Around coasts of Britain.
Appearance	A large trailing seaweed, dark green in colour.
Part used	Dried plant.
Therapeutic uses	Acts on thyroid. Tones up the system and clears the kidneys.
Prepared as	Decoction. An ointment is used in psoriasis.

Blue Flag
IRIS VERSICOLOR

Also known as	Flag Lily or Water Flag.
Where found	Extensively planted in gardens throughout Britain.
Appearance	A beautiful plant with arching strap-like leaves and blue, white, yellow or multi-coloured flowers.

40

Part used	Rhizome.
Therapeutic uses	Principally used as a blood purifier. Also an alterative, diuretic and cathartic. Indicated in skin diseases.
Prepared as	Decoction.

Boldo
PEUMUS BOLDUS

Also known as	Boldu.
Found wild	Chile.
Appearance	Medium-size shrub with dark oval leaves and a strong lemon smell.
Part used	Leaves.
Therapeutic uses	Used as a liver stimulant. It also has antiseptic properties and is of value to sufferers of catarrh of the bladder.
Prepared as	Decoction.

Borage
BORAGO OFFICINALIS

Also known as	Burrage.
Found wild	Throughout Europe.
Appearance	Bold, erect herb of strong growth with small blue flowers.
Part used	Leaves.
Therapeutic uses	As a tonic and stimulant, also as a remedy for migraine and headaches. Poultice for inflammations.
Prepared as	Decoction.

Bugloss
Echium vulgare

Also known as	Viper's Bugloss.
Found wild	Europe.
Appearance	A sturdy herb with blue flowers.
Part used	Herb.
Therapeutic uses	An expectorant and demulcent. Excellent for gentle bowel action. Also to clear phlegm from bronchial tubes.
Prepared as	Infusion.

Burdock
ARCTIUM LAPPA

Also known as	Cockle Buttons.
Found wild	UK and Europe.
Appearance	Strong-growing plant with large leaves.
Part used	Root, seeds and leaves.
Therapeutic uses	Diuretic and diaphoretic. For skin eruptions, psoriasis, eczema and rheumatic complaints.
Prepared as	Infusion or decoction.

Bush Tea
CYCLOPIA GENISTOIDES

Also known as	Red Bush.
Found wild	South Africa.

Appearance	Small erect bush of striking appearance.
Part used	Herb.
Therapeutic uses	For kidney and liver disorders.
Prepared as	Infusion.

Canella
CANELLA ALBA

Also known as	Wild Cinnamon.
Found wild	West Indies.
Appearance	Slender branching tree with light grey bark.
Part used	Bark.
Therapeutic uses	Stimulant tonic for the aged. Promotes digestion and elimination and prevents flatulence.
Prepared as	Decoction.

Caraway
CARUM CARVI

Also known as	Caraway Seed.
Found wild	Europe and North Africa.
Appearance	A hollow-stemmed herb.
Part used	Fruit.
Therapeutic uses	As a flavouring.
Prepared as	Decoction or powder.

Burdock Root
ARCTIUM LAPPA

Also known as	Cockle Buttons.
Found wild	UK and Europe.
Appearance	Strong-growing plant with large leaves.
Parts used	Roots, seeds and leaves.
Therapeutic uses	Diuretic and diaphoretic, used for skin eruptions, acne, psoriasis, eczema and rheumatic problems.
Prepared as	Infusion or decoction.

Bush Tea
CYCLOPIA GENISTOIDES

Also known as	Red Bush.
Found wild	South Africa.
Appearance	Small, erect bush of striking appearance.
Part used	Herb.
Therapeutic uses	For kidney and liver disorders.
Prepared as	Infusion.

Cajuput
MELALEUCA LEUCADENDRON

Also known as	White Tea Tree.
Found wild	East Indies.
Appearance	A large tree.
Part used	Oil.

Therapeutic uses	Treatment of rheumatism, bruises and sprains.
Prepared as	Lotion or ointments.

Canella
CANELLA ALBA

Also known as	Wild Cinnamon.
Found wild	West Indies.
Appearance	Slender branching tree with light grey bark.
Part used	Bark.
Therapeutic uses	Stimulant tonic for the aged. Promotes digestion and elimination and prevents flatulence.
Prepared as	Decoction.

Caroba
JACARANDA PROCERA

Also known as	Carob Tree.
Found wild	South Africa and South America.
Appearance	A handsome tree with lanceolate leaves.
Part used	Leaves.
Therapeutic uses	As a diaphoretic and diuretic. Also as a sedative.
Prepared as	Infusion.

Chamomile, Belgian
ANTHEMIS NOBILIS

Found wild	Belgium and France. Widely cultivated.
Appearance	Herb with double flowers.
Part used	Flowers.
Therapeutic uses	Widely used for women suffering from nervous upsets and as a tonic, stomachic and antispasmodic.
Prepared as	Infusion.

Chamomile, German
MATRICARIA CHAMOMILLA

Found wild	Europe.
Appearance	Herb with small cushion-like flowers in profusion.
Part used	Flowers.
Therapeutic uses	Excellent nerve sedative, carminative and tonic and as a poultice for leg ulcers.
Prepared as	Infusion and poultice.

Chickweed
STELLARIA MEDIA

Also known as	Starweed.
Found wild	Britain.
Appearance	Small prolific weed.

Part used	Herb.
Therapeutic uses	A demulcent and to allay feverish conditions.
Prepared as	Decoction.

Chiretta
SWERTIA CHIRATA

Also known as	Indian Gentian.
Found wild	India.
Appearance	Small wiry herb growing in arid places.
Part used	Herb.
Therapeutic uses	Tonic to restore flagging appetite.
Prepared as	Decoction.

Clover, Red
TRIFOLIUM PRATENSE

Also known as	Trefoil.
Found wild	Throughout Europe.
Appearance	A common clover.
Part used	Herb.
Therapeutic uses	Used as a sedative and to clear up nervous coughs, 'tickling' coughs and whooping cough. It is one of the best herbs to use for children.
Prepared as	Infusion.

Appearance	Small prolific weed.
Part used	Herb.
Therapeutic uses	A demulcent and to allay feverish conditions. Soothing to the skin.
Prepared as	Decoction and ointment.

Chiretta
SWERTIA CHIRATA

Also known as	Indian Gentian.
Found wild	India.
Appearance	Small, wiry herb which grows in arid places.
Part used	Plant.
Therapeutic uses	Tonic to restore flagging appetite.
Prepared as	Decoction.

Clivers
GALIUM APARINE

Also known as	Goosegrass.
Found wild	UK.
Appearance	Strong-growing weed.
Part used	Herb.
Therapeutic uses	Diuretic, aperient. Also for psoriasis.
Prepared as	Infusion.

Cloves
EUGENIA CARYOPHYLLUS

Found wild	Zanzibar, Madagascar and East Indies.
Appearance	Beautiful evergreen tree of majestic appearance.
Part used	Flower, buds and oil.
Therapeutic uses	A stimulant and carminative, usually compounded with other remedies.
Prepared as	Decoction.

Clubmoss
LYCOPODIUM CLAVATUM

Found wild	Northern hemisphere.
Appearance	Low spreading greyish/green plant usually found near water.
Part used	Plant.
Therapeutic uses	Treatment of cystitis, kidney complaints and urinary disorders. Also a sedative and for stomach disorders.
Prepared as	Infusion.

Cohosh (Blue)
CAULOPHYLLUM THALICTROIDES

Also known as	Blueberry Root.
Found wild	United States and Canada.
Appearance	A gnarled, crowded shrub.
Part used	Rhizome.

Cornsilk
ZEA MAYS

Found wild	South Africa and America.
Appearance	Maize.
Part used	Part of flower.
Therapeutic uses	Principally as a diuretic but also for pulmonary troubles.
Prepared as	Decoction.

Cotton Root
GOSSYPIUM HERBACEUM

Found wild	Mediterranean islands and the United States.
Appearance	Twist of bark.
Part used	Bark of root.
Therapeutic uses	Treatment of women's disorders.
Prepared as	Infusion.

Cowslip
PRIMULA OFFICINALIS

Also known as	Paigle.
Found wild	UK and Europe.
Appearance	Small wild flower.
Part used	Flowers.
Therapeutic uses	Sedative and hypnotic. Helpful in cases of insomnia and nervous restlessness.
Prepared as	Infusion.

Cramp Bark
VIBURNUM OPULUS

Also known as	Snow-ball Tree, Guelder Rose.
Found wild	Europe and America.
Appearance	Strong-growing bush with white ball-shaped flowers.
Part used	Bark.
Therapeutic uses	As a nervine for treatment of spasms and convulsions. Antispasmodic. Regarded as a safe children's medication.
Prepared as	Decoction.

Cranesbill, American
GERANIUM MACULATUM

Also known as	Wild Geranium, Storksbill.
Found wild	United States.
Appearance	Shrubby small herb with blue flowers.
Parts used	Herb and root.
Therapeutic uses	Has quick styptic properties and is a tonic and astringent. Used as a treatment for piles and ulcers.
Prepared as	Decoction.

Parts used	Herb. Root.
Therapeutic uses	Has quick styptic properties and is a tonic and astringent. Used as a treatment for piles and ulcers.
Prepared as	Decoction.

Dandelion
TARAXACUM OFFICINALE

Appearance	Common herb with long root, toothed leaves and bright yellow flowers.
Parts used	Leaves and root.
Therapeutic uses	As a tonic and diuretic and for liver and kidney ills. Roots frequently used for coffee as they contain no caffeine.
Prepared as	Decoction or infusion.

Dodder
CUSCUTA EPITHYMUM

Found wild	Throughout the world.
Appearance	A climbing parasite of the convolvulus family.
Part used	Herb.
Therapeutic uses	As a mild laxative and hepatic, for the treatment of bladder and liver troubles.
Prepared as	Infusion.

Dog Rose
ROSA CANINA

Also known as	Wild Briar.
Found wild	Europe and Middle East.
Appearance	The wild rose.
Part used	Fruit.
Therapeutic uses	The fruit yields ascorbic acid (vitamin C) of great value when given to young children.
Prepared as	Syrup.

Echinacea
ECHINACEA ANGUSTIFOLIA

Also known as	Coneflower.
Found wild	United States.
Appearance	Herb of medium height.
Part used	Rhizome.
Therapeutic uses	Antiseptic and alterative. Helps to purify the blood. Useful for boils and carbuncles.
Prepared as	Decoction.

Elder
SAMBUCUS NIGRA

Also known as	Black Elder.
Found wild	Europe.
Appearance	A tall straggling shrub with profuse crops of black berries.
Parts used	Flowers, berries and bark.

Elder
SAMBUCUS NIGRA

Also known as	Black Elder.
Found wild	Europe.
Appearance	A tall straggling shrub with profuse crops of black berries.
Parts used	Flowers, berries and bark.
Therapeutic uses	For colds and influenza. As an alterative and diuretic. It is a safe soporific and induces healthy sleep.
Prepared as	Infusion.

Evening Primrose
OENOTHERA BIENNIS

Also known as	Tree Primrose.
Found wild	European gardens.
Appearance	Small herb with a delightful display of yellow flowers.
Parts used	Leaves and bark.
Therapeutic uses	As a sedative and astringent. For the relief of female menstrual disorders.
Prepared as	Decoction. The oil of evening primrose is now extensively used.

Fenugreek
TRIGONELLA FOENUM-GRAECUM

Found wild	Mediterranean area, North Africa and India.

Appearance	Slender-stemmed plant.
Part used	Herb.
Therapeutic uses	As an emolient, a laxative and expectorant. Can be applied externally to assist gout, ulcers, wounds and boils.
Prepared as	Decoction and poultice.

Feverfew
TANACETUM PARTHENIUM

Also known as	Featherfew.
Found wild	Throughout Europe.
Appearance	A small grey herb with hairy stems.
Part used	Herb.
Therapeutic uses	As an aperient, also used by women to bring on the menses. An effective remedy for migraine.
Prepared as	Infusion.

Figwort
SCROPHULARIA NODOSA

| **Also known as** | Throatwort. |
| **Found wild** | Throughout Europe. |

Appearance	A small tree with inconspicuous white flowers and a very bitter taste.
Part used	The bark of the root.
Therapeutic uses	Tonic, alterative and diuretic. Also treatment of liver disorders, gallstones and jaundice.
Prepared as	Decoction.

Fumitory
FUMARIA OFFICINALIS

Found wild	Europe.
Appearance	A small low-growing herb.
Parts used	Stem and leaves.
Therapeutic uses	Gentle aperient and diuretic. Used to bathe skin eruptions.
Prepared as	Infusion.

Garlic
ALLIUM SATIVUM

Where found	Universally cultivated.
Appearance	Similar to shallot.
Part used	Bulb.
Therapeutic uses	Antifungal. For treatment of dyspepsia and flatulence. Also as a stimulant.
Prepared as	Juice or tincture.

Gentian
GENTIANA LUTEA

Found wild	Mountain meadows of Europe.
Appearance	A plant with oblong, pale green leaves and large yellow scented flowers.
Part used	Root.
Therapeutic use	Tonic.
Prepared as	Decoction or powder.

Germander
TEUCRIUM CHAMAEDRYS

Also known as	Wall Germander.
Found wild	UK and Europe.
Appearance	Stemmed plant growing to 61 cm/ 2 feet.
Part used	Herb.
Therapeutic uses	A helpful plant for the treatment of rheumatoid arthritis and gout. Has anti-inflammatory properties.
Prepared as	Decoction.

Ginger
ZINGIBER OFFICINALE

Found wild	West Indies and China.
Appearance	Height, about 91 cm/3 feet with glossy aromatic leaves.
Part used	Rhizome.

| **Therapeutic uses** | Has stimulative and carminative properties and can be used as an expectorant and an aid to digestion. |
| **Prepared as** | Powder or decoction. |

Ginseng
PANAX QUINQUEFOLIUM

Also known as	Panax.
Found wild	China and Mongolia.
Appearance	Erect-growing herb with fleshy leaves.
Part used	Root.
Therapeutic uses	Sedative, stomachic and tonic. Improves fertility.
Prepared as	Decoction.

Golden Seal
HYDRASTIS CANADENSIS

Also known as	Yellow Root.
Where found	Cultivated in North America.
Appearance	Tall-growing herb with disagreeable odour.
Part used	Rhizome.
Therapeutic uses	For gastric disorders and as a soothing laxative and tonic.
Prepared as	Decoction or powder.

Guarana
PAULPINIA CUPANA

Also known as	Brazilian Cocoa.
Found wild	Brazil.
Appearance	A tall arching shrub.
Part used	Seeds.
Therapeutic uses	As a stimulant and for relief of headaches and migraine. Also used by women to bring on the menses and can be effective in the treatment of arthritis.
Prepared as	Decoction or powder.

Hawthorn
CRATAEGUS OXYCANTHA

Also known as	May Tree.
Found wild	Throughout Britain.
Appearance	A common small tree.
Part used	Fruit.
Therapeutic use	A good general heart tonic.
Prepared as	Decoction.

Holy Thistle
CARBENIA BENEDICTA

Also known as	Blessed Thistle
Found wild	Southern Europe.
Appearance	Typical thistle.
Part used	Stem and leaves.

Part used	Stem and leaves.
Therapeutic uses	A safe emmenagogue and diaphoretic. Helpful externally for ulcers.
Prepared as	Infusion.

Hops
HUMULUS LUPULUS

Found wild	Europe. Cultivated in most parts of the world.
Appearance	A climbing vine.
Part used	Strobiles.
Therapeutic uses	As an anodyne for the relief of pain. Also as a tonic and an aid for stomach disorders and to promote sleep.
Prepared as	Infusion.

Horseradish
COCHLEARIA ARMORACIA

Found wild	Europe.
Appearance	A herb growing to 91 cm/3 feet, with a pungent odour.
Part used	Root.
Therapeutic uses	Relieves flatulence and indigestion. Promotes perspiration and is a diuretic.
Prepared as	Infusion.

Horsetail
EQUISETUM ARVENSE

Also known as	Scouring Rushes.
Found wild	Great Britain.
Appearance	A tall, bold herb with cane-like appearance.
Part used	Herb.
Therapeutic uses	A powerful astringent and also a diuretic. Excellent for kidney troubles.
Prepared as	Decoction.

Houndstongue
CYNOGLOSSUM OFFICINALE

Found wild	Great Britain.
Appearance	A medium-sized herb with long, straplike leaves.
Part used	Herb.
Therapeutic uses	An anodyne for relief of pain. Also as a demulcent for soothing coughs and colds. Can also be used to reduce piles.
Prepared as	Infusion.

Houseleek
SEMPERVIVUM TECTORUM

Found wild	Throughout Great Britain.
Appearance	A small procumbent plant.

Hyssop
HYSSOPUS OFFICINALIS

Found wild	UK.
Appearance	Small common field herb.
Part used	Leaves.
Therapeutic uses	Stimulant and carminative for bronchial and nasal catarrh. Also for anxiety states and tension.
Prepared as	Infusion.

Iceland Moss
CETRARIA ISLANDICA

Found wild	Throughout northern hemisphere.
Appearance	This is not a moss but a procumbent grey lichen.
Part used	Plant.
Therapeutic uses	For catarrh and bronchitis. It is a nutritive and helpful for digestive disorders.
Prepared as	Decoction.

Jaborandi
PILOCARPUS MICROPHYLLUS

Found wild	Brazil.
Appearance	A small herb.

Part used	Leaves.
Therapeutic uses	A diaphoretic and expectorant and is beneficial to asthma sufferers.
Prepared as	Decoction — external use only. Restricted purchase only. Usually sold as one part Jaborandi to 19 parts Rosemary.

Jalap
IPOMAEGA PURGA

Found wild	South America.
Appearance	A robust climbing plant.
Part used	Root.
Therapeutic use	Strong laxative, combine with ginger.
Prepared as	Decoction.

Jambul
EUGENIA JAMBOLANA

Also known as	Java Plum.
Found wild	East India.
Appearance	A large spreading tree.
Part used	Seeds.
Therapeutic uses	Helpful to diabetics. Reduces sugar content of urine.
Prepared as	Decoction.

Jambul
EUGENIA JAMBOLANA

Also known as	Java Plum.
Found wild	East India.
Appearance	A large spreading tree.
Part used	Seeds.
Therapeutic uses	Helpful for diabetics. Quickly reduces urinal sugar content.
Prepared as	Decoction.

Kava
PIPER METHYSTICUM

Also known as	Kava-Kava.
Found wild	South Pacific.
Appearance	Tall shrub.
Part used	Root.
Therapeutic uses	As a tonic and as a diuretic. Helpful for the treatment of joint pains, rheumatism and gout.
Prepared as	Decoction.

Lady's Mantle
ALCHEMILLA VULGARIS

Also known as	Lion's Foot.
Found wild	UK.
Appearance	Low-growing herb with small green flowers.
Part used	Leaves.

| **Therapeutic uses** | Allays menstrual flooding. Also astyptic and astringent. Externally used as a douche for pruritis vulvae. |
| **Prepared as** | Infusion. |

Lettuce (Wild)
LACTUCA VIROSA

Found wild	Warm parts of Europe.
Appearance	A small plant of bushy appearance.
Parts used	Leaves and juice.
Therapeutic uses	An anodyne and sedative. Also useful for easing coughs of nervous origin. Relieves rheumatic pain.
Prepared as	Decoction.

Lime Flowers
TILIA EUROPOEA

Also known as	Linden Flowers.
Found wild	Throughout Europe.
Appearance	A graceful tree.
Part used	Flowers.
Therapeutic uses	A strong, but safe, nervine for relief of headaches and hysteria. Also a stimulant and tonic.
Prepared as	Infusion.

Lime Flowers
TILIA EUROPOEA

Also known as	Linden Flowers.
Found wild	Throughout Europe.
Appearance	A graceful tree.
Part used	Flowers.
Therapeutic uses	A strong but safe nervine for relief of headaches and hysteria. Also as a stimulant and tonic.
Prepared as	Infusion.

Liquorice
GLYCYRRHIZA GLABRA

Found wild	Europe and the Middle East.
Appearance	A strong-growing perennial plant.
Part used	Root.
Therapeutic uses	In cough medicines. As a demulcent and pectoral and as a gentle laxative.
Prepared as	Decoction.

Logwood
HAEMATOXYLON CAMPECHIANUM

Found wild	South America.
Appearance	A massive tree.
Part used	Wood.
Therapeutic uses	To relieve diarrhoea and dysentery. Also helpful for women's disorders.
Prepared as	Decoction.

Manna
FRAXINUS ORNUS

Found wild	Mediterranean countries.
Appearance	Medium-sized shrub.
Part used	Sap from cuts in bark.
Therapeutic uses	As a gentle laxative for pregnant women and as a nutritive invalid food.
Prepared as	Decoction.

Marshmallow
ALTHAEA OFFICINALIS

Found wild	Throughout Europe.
Appearance	A strong-growing herb usually found in watery places.
Parts used	Leaves and root.
Therapeutic uses	As an emollient and demulcent for incorporation in cough medicines. Also for treatment of cystitis and for soothing the alimentary canal.
Prepared as	Infusion and poultice.

Mayweed
ANTHEMIS COTULA

Also known as	Dog Fennel.
Found wild	Throughout Europe.
Appearance	A low-growing herb and common weed.
Part used	Herb.

Marshmallow
ALTHAEA OFFICINALIS

Found wild	Throughout Europe.
Appearance	A strong-growing herb, usually found in watery places.
Part used	Leaves.
Therapeutic uses	As an emollient and demulcent for incorporation in cough medicines. Also for treatment of cystitis and for soothing the alimentary canal.
Prepared as	Infusion or poultice.

Marshmallow Root
ALTHAEA OFFICINALIS

Also known as	Guimauve.
Found wild	Europe and UK.
Appearance	Strong-growing herb, often found near water.
Parts used	Roots and leaves.
Therapeutic uses	A demulcent, emollient and diuretic. Also used as a poultice for skin ulcers and general inflammation.
Prepared as	Decoction, poultice or ointment.

Mayweed
ANTHEMIS COTULA

Also known as	Dog Fennel.
Found wild	Throughout Europe.
Appearance	A low-growing herb which is a common weed.
Part used	Herb.
Therapeutic uses	An antispasmodic with marked tonic qualities. Excellent for migraine.
Prepared as	Infusion.

Meadowsweet
FILIPENDULA ULMARIA

Also known as	Bridewort.
Found wild	UK and Europe.
Appearance	Long-stemmed herb growing to 1.5 m/5 feet.
Part used	Herb.
Therapeutic uses	An anti-rheumatic, stomachic and astringent. Helpful for severe cases of cystitis, muscular rheumatic and joint pains.
Prepared as	Infusion.

Motherwort
LEONURUS CARDIACA

Where found	A common garden plant in Britain and northern Europe.

| **Therapeutic uses** | Carminative, anti-emetic. Helpful in most cases of stomach upset. Can be used externally for the treatment of rheumatic pain. *Use in moderation*. |
| **Prepared as** | Powder and oil. |

Oats
AVENA SATIVA

Found wild	In most temperate climates.
Appearance	A common farm crop similar to wheat.
Part used	Seeds.
Therapeutic uses	An effective nerve tonic and to allay spasms. Relieves rheumatic pain.
Prepared as	Decoction.

Papaw
CARICA PAPAYA

Also known as	Melon Tree.
Found wild	Throughout sub-tropical areas.
Appearance	A tall tree (about seven metres) with boldly serrated leaves. only the female produces fruit.
Part used	Papain from the juice.
Therapeutic uses	As a digestive aid, helpful for duodenal and peptic ulcers.
Prepared as	Powder.

Paraguay Tea
ILEX PARAGUENSIS

Also known as	Mate Tea.
Found wild	South America.
Appearance	A dense shrub.
Part used	Leaves.
Therapeutic uses	Stimulant. Very helpful in the relief of rheumatism and arthritis. Commonly used to make a pleasant tea.
Prepared as	Infusion.

Parsley
CARUM PETROSELINUM

Found wild	Europe.
Appearance	Bienniel umbelliferous plant with white flowers and aromatic leaves.
Parts used	Seeds, root and leaves.
Therapeutic uses	As a diuretic and in the treatment of kidney disorders, stones and gravel. Emmenagogue and in the treatment of amenorrhoea.
Prepared as	Decoction.

Parsley Piert
ALCHEMILLA ARVENSIS

Also known as	Beakstone.
Found wild	Throughout Europe.

Oats
AVENA SATIVA

Found wild	In most temperate climates.
Appearance	A common farm crop similar to wheat.
Part used	Seeds.
Therapeutic uses	An effective nerve tonic. Also allays spasms and relieves rheumatic pain.
Prepared as	Decoction.

Papaw
CARICA PAPAYA

Also known as	Melon Tree.
Found wild	Throughout sub-tropical areas.
Appearance	A tall tree (about 8 m/25 feet) with boldly-serrated leaves. Only the female produces fruit.
Part used	Papain from the juice.
Therapeutic uses	As a digestive aid, helpful for duodenal and peptic ulcers.
Prepared as	Powder.

Paraguay Tea
ILEX PARAQUENSIS

Also known as	Mate Tea.
Found wild	South America.
Appearance	A dense shrub.
Part used	Leaves.

| **Therapeutic uses** | Stimulant. Very helpful in the relief of rheumatism and arthritis. Commonly used to make a pleasant tea. |
| **Prepared as** | Infusion. |

Parsley
CARUM PETROSELINUM

Found wild	Europe.
Appearance	Biennial umbelliferous plant with white flowers and aromatic leaves.
Parts used	Seeds, root and leaves.
Therapeutic uses	Used as a diuretic and in the treatment of kidney disorders, stones and gravel. Also as an emmenagogue and in the treatment of amenorrhoea.
Prepared as	Decoction.

Parsley Piert
ALCHEMILLA ARVENSIS

Also known as	Beakstone.
Found wild	Throughout Europe.
Appearance	A low-growing herb with tiny green flowers. Not related to common parsley.
Part used	Herb.
Therapeutic uses	For the relief of bladder and kidney troubles, and helpful in dissolving kidney stones.

Part used	Herb.
Therapeutic uses	Stomachic and carminative. Relieves sickness, flatulence and indigestion.
Prepared as	Infusion.

Periwinkle, South African
VINCA ROSA

Found wild	South Africa.
Appearance	Large trailing herb with profuse pink flowers.
Part used	Herb.
Therapeutic uses	Helpful for treatment of diabetes.
Prepared as	Infusion.

Pichi
FABIANA IMBRICATA

Found wild	South America.
Appearance	Herb of moderate growth with tiny leaves.
Parts used	Leaves and wood.
Therapeutic uses	Hepatic. Recommended for treatment of liver disorders. Also a stimulant and diuretic and helpful for catarrhal and kidney troubles.
Prepared as	Infusion.

Pilewort
RANUNCULUS FICARIA

Also known as	Lesser Celandine.
Found wild	UK and Europe.
Appearance	A procumbent yellow-flowered herb.
Part used	Herb.
Therapeutic uses	Excellent for treatment of piles.
Prepared as	Infusion and ointment.

Poplar, White
POPULUS TREMULOIDES

Found wild	UK and Europe.
Appearance	Large tree.
Part used	Bark.
Therapeutic uses	Anti-rheumatic. Anti-inflammatory. Antiseptic. Beneficial to all cases of muscular and arthritic rheumatism.
Prepared as	Decoction.

Prickly Ash
XANTHOXYLUM CLAVANERCULIS

Found wild	North America.
Appearance	Medium-sized tree.
Parts used	Bark and berries.

Pichi
FABIANA IMBRICATA

Found wild	South America.
Appearance	Herb of moderate growth with tiny leaves.
Parts used	Leaves and wood.
Therapeutic uses	A hepatic, recommended for treatment of liver disorders. Also a stimulant and diuretic and helpful for catarrhal and kidney troubles.
Prepared as	Infusion.

Pilewort
RANUNCULUS FICARIA

Also known as	Lesser Celandine.
Found wild	Europe and UK.
Appearance	A procumbent yellow-flowered herb.
Part used	Herb.
Therapeutic use	Excellent for treatment of piles.
Prepared as	Infusion or ointment.

Poke Root
PHYTOLACCA DECANDRA

Found wild	North America.
Appearance	Shrub with grape-sized black berries.

Parts used	Root and berries.
Therapeutic uses	An emetic, cathartic and anti-rheumatic. External application for skin eruptions such as acne.
Prepared as	Infusion or ointment.

Prickly Ash Bark
ZANTHOXYLUM AMERICANUM

Found wild	North America.
Appearance	Medium-sized tree.
Parts used	Bark and berries.
Therapeutic uses	A diaphoretic, carminative and stimulant. Helpful for circulation disorders associated with rheumatism.
Prepared as	Decoction.

Pulsatilla
ANEMONE PULSATILLA

Also known as	Wind Flower.
Found wild	Europe and UK.
Appearance	A large weed with purple flowers.
Part used	Leaves.
Therapeutic uses	A sedative, nervine and antispasmodic. Helpful for women with menstrual problems. Also used for headaches associated with tension, insomnia and skin eruptions.
Prepared as	Infusion (dried herb only).

Therapeutic uses	Carminative, nervine, tonic. Helpful in cases of tension and migraine headaches. Associated with hair care.
Prepared as	Infusion.

St John's Wort
HYPERICUM PERFORATUM

Found wild	Britain.
Appearance	Sturdy yellow-flowered herb.
Part used	Herb.
Therapeutic uses	Diuretic. Expectorant, helpful for coughs and bronchial ailments.
Prepared as	Decoction.

Samphire
CRITHMUM MARITIMUM

Also known as	Rock Samphire.
Found wild	England, particularly in saline conditions.
Appearance	A small herb that prefers shelter of rocks.
Part used	Herb.
Therapeutic uses	Diuretic with a beneficial kidney action. Helpful for weight loss.
Prepared as	Infusion.

Sarsparilla
SMILAX MEDICA

Found wild	South America.
Appearance	Bush.
Part used	Rhizome.
Therapeutic uses	Alterative, anti-rheumatic, antiseptic. Helpful in cases of psoriasis and other skin ailments. Long standing treatment for severe rheumatism and rheumatoid arthritis.
Prepared as	Decoction.

Savory, Summer
SATUREIA HORTENSIS

Where found	Commonly cultivated throughout the world.
Appearance	A small shrubby plant.
Part used	Herb.
Therapeutic uses	For relief of flatulence and indigestion. Also as a poultice to reduce inflammations.
Prepared as	Decoction.

Scullcap
SCUTELLARIA LATERIFOLIA

Found wild	United States.
Appearance	A herb of insignificant appearance with pale blue flowers.
Part used	Herb.

Found wild	England, particularly in saline conditions.
Appearance	A small herb that prefers the shelter of rocks.
Part used	Herb.
Therapeutic uses	A diuretic with a beneficial kidney action. Helpful for weight loss.
Prepared as	Infusion.

Sarsaparilla
SMILAX ORNATA

Also known as	Jamaican Sarsaparilla.
Found wild	Caribbean and Central America.
Appearance	Shrub.
Part used	Root.
Therapeutic uses	An alterative, blood purifier and antiseptic. Externally of great benefit to psoriasis sufferers.
Prepared as	Infusion.

Savory (Summer)
SATUREIA HORTENSIS

Where found	Commonly cultivated throughout the world.
Appearance	A small shrubby plant.
Part used	Herb.
Therapeutic uses	For relief of flatulence and indigestion. Also as a poultice to reduce inflammations.
Prepared as	Decoction.

Senna
CASSIA AUGUSTIFOLIA

Found wild	Arabia.
Appearance	Tree of sparse growth with distinctive grey/green leaves.
Parts used	Leaves and seed case.
Therapeutic uses	Laxative.
Prepared as	Infusion.

Shepherd's Purse
CAPSELLA BURSA-PASTORIS

Found wild	Everywhere.
Appearance	Small insignificant weed with little white flowers.
Part used	Herb.
Therapeutic uses	Diuretic, usually for kidney and urinary troubles. Also an antiscorbutic.
Prepared as	Infusion.

Slippery Elm
ULMUS FULVA

Found wild	North America.
Appearance	A great tree of spreading growth.
Part used	Inner part of bark.
Therapeutic uses	As a nutritive for invalids. Also as an emollient and demulcent for healing burns and skin troubles.

Squill
URFINEA MARITIMA

Found wild	Southern Europe and North Africa.
Appearance	One of the lily family.
Part used	Corm.
Therapeutic uses	One of the most beneficial and much used herbs. Expectorant. Helpful in relieving catarrh, asthma and bronchial troubles. Also a cathartic and diuretic.
Prepared as	Decoction.

Swamp Milkweed
ASCLEPIAS INCARNATA

Found wild	United States.
Appearance	Medium-sized shrub of grotesque appearance.
Parts used	Rhizome and root.
Therapeutic uses	It is a cathartic and an emetic. Beneficial in the treatment of arthritis and stomach disorders.
Prepared as	Infusion.

Sweet Chestnut
CASTANEA SATIVA

Found wild	UK and Europe.
Appearance	Large tree.
Part used	Leaves.

Therapeutic uses	Astringent. Anti-rheumatic. Helpful in cases of muscular rheumatism, lumbago and fibrositis. Of specific benefit to catarrhal conditions.
Prepared as	Infusion.

Sweet Sumach
RHUS AROMATICA

Where found	Canada and the United States.
Appearance	A shrub growing to about 4ft high.
Part used	Root-bark.
Therapeutic uses	Astringent and diuretic used in the treatment of incontinence in children and in the elderly.
Prepared as	Infusion.

Thuja
THUJA OCCIDENTALIS

Also known as	Tree of life, yellow cedar.
Where found	Canada and the United States.
Appearance	A coniferous tree.
Part used	Leaves.
Therapeutic uses	Expectorant and emmenagogue, used in coughs, absence of menstrual periods and gout. Used externally as a lotion for the removal of warts.
Prepared as	Cold infusion, taken in tablespoonful doses.

Thuja
THUJA OCCIDENTALIS

Also known as	Arbor Vitae.
Found wild	Canada and USA.
Appearance	Spreading conifer of small size.
Part used	Leaves.
Therapeutic uses	Used externally as lotion for psoriasis, eczema and warts.
Prepared as	Infusion, lotion or tincture.

Thyme
THYMUS VULGARIS

Where found	Common garden plant.
Appearance	Small perennial herb with tiny leaves.
Part used	Herb.
Therapeutic uses	Antispasmodic and tonic. Contains thymol, a strong antiseptic, useful in irritable coughs and catarrh.
Prepared as	Infusion is sweetened with honey and given in tablespoonful doses.

Water Betony
SCROPHULARIA AQUATICA

Also known as	Brown Wort.

Found wild	Europe and UK.
Appearance	Medium-sized herb with an affinity for water.
Part used	Leaves.
Therapeutic uses	A vulnerary. Also excellent for skin complaints.
Prepared as	Poultice or ointment.

Water Dock
RUMEX AQUATICUS

Also known as	Bloodwort.
Found wild	Throughout Europe.
Appearance	One of the common dock family.
Part used	Root.
Therapeutic uses	An alterative and detergent. It helps clean and strengthen gums and relieves mouth ulcers.
Prepared as	Infusion.

White Poplar
POPULUS TREMULOIDES

Found wild	UK and Europe.
Appearance	Large tree.
Part used	Bark.
Therapeutic uses	An anti-rheumatic, anti-inflammatory and antiseptic. It is beneficial in all cases of muscular and arthritic rheumatism.

Wild Yam
DIOSCOREA VILLOSA

Also known as	Rheumatism Root and Colic Root.
Found wild	North America and tropical areas.
Appearance	Tuberous plant.
Part used	Root.
Therapeutic uses	Anti-inflammatory, antispasmodic, diaphoretic. Helpful in the treatment of rheumatoid arthritis and muscular rheumatism. Leg cramps and intermittent claudication are two other conditions which can be beneficially treated.
Prepared as	Decoction.

Wood Sage
TEUCRIUM SCORODONIA

Also known as	Garlic Sage.
Found wild	UK.
Appearance	Small herb.
Part used	Herb.
Therapeutic uses	Respiratory infections, astringent, anti-rheumatic. This herb has been used for many years to treat respiratory infections and also rheumatic pain and stiffness.
Prepared as	Infusion.

Yarrow
ACHILLEA MILLEFOLIUM

Also known as	Milfoil.
Found wild	Britain.
Appearance	A tiny herb.
Part used	Herb.
Therapeutic uses	A stimulant and diaphoretic. Excellent for treatment of influenza and heavy chest colds.
Prepared as	Infusion.

Part used	Herb.
Therapeutic uses	A stimulant and diaphoretic which is excellent for the treatment of influenza and heavy chest colds. Helpful for blood purifying.
Prepared as	Infusion.

Yellow Dock Root
RUMEX CRISPUS

Also known as	Curled Dock Root.
Found wild	UK.
Appearance	Common weed with long narrow leaves.
Part used	Root.
Therapeutic uses	A laxative and cholagogue. Also used for skin diseases, particularly where constipation is a problem.
Prepared as	Decoction.

A guide to
herbal suppliers

Medical herbalists practise in most towns, while health food shops should be able to assist with the more common dried herbs. Specialist requirements, though, often need specialist stockists.

The following list is by no means complete, but should be sufficient to cover most herbs mentioned in this book.

MAIL ORDER STOCKISTS

Cathay of Bournemouth Ltd
3 Wickham Road
Bournemouth
Dorset
BH7 6JX
(Free literature on request.)

Culpeper Ltd
Hadstock Road
Linton
Cambs
CB1 6NJ

MAJOR RETAIL OUTLETS

Bournemouth Cathay of Bournemouth Ltd
3 Wickham Road
Bournemouth
Dorset
BH7 6JX

Gerard House
736 Christchurch Road
Bournemouth,
and

31 St Thomas Street
Lymington
Hants

Edinburgh   Napiers of Edinburgh
18 Bristo Place
Edinburgh
EH1 1EZ

London   G. Baldwin
173 Walworth Road
London
SE17 1RW

Neal's Yard Remedies
Neal's Yard
Covent Garden
London
WC2H 9DP

Ryde   The Grail
1 The High Street
Ryde
Isle of Wight
PO33 2PN

Culpeper Herbal Shops can be found in nine major towns, including three in London.

A directory of medical herbalists is available from the National Institute of Medical Herbalists, 9 Palace Gate, Exeter, Devon, EX1 1JA. It is advisable to consult a medical herbalist if any doubt exists about a particular condition or suggested remedy.

Glossary of common medical terms

Very often when reading, or on having a medical consultation, words are used which may not be familiar. This short list will help to make some of the more common ones a little clearer.

Alterative   Any substance that can beneficially alter the condition of a patient.

Amenorrhoea   Cessation of the menstrual flow.

Anodyne   Any substance which eases pain.

Antiseptic   Any substance that prevents putrefaction.

Antispasmodic   Any substance that prevents or relieves spasms.

Anthelmintic   Any herb acting against intestinal worms.

Aperient   Any substance producing the natural evacuation of the bowels.

Aphrodisiac   Any substance that stimulates sexual functions.

| **Astringent** | Any substance which causes contraction of body tissues. |

Cardiac Any condition affecting or pertaining to the heart.

Carminative Any substance that relieves pain caused by flatulence.

Cathartic Any substance that induces stimulation of bowel action; rather stronger than aperients.

Corrective Any substance that restores normal conditions.

Debility Feebleness of health.

Degenerative Deterioration or change in tissue structure.

Demulcent Any soothing medicine.

Deobstruent Any substance that frees the natural orifices of the body.

Diaphoretic Any substance inducing perspiration.

Diuretic Any substance that increases the flow of urine.

Dysmenorrhoea Excessive pain during menstruation.

Emetic	Any substance that causes vomiting.
Emmenagogue	Any drug that stimulates menstruation.
Emollient	Any substance that soothes and lubricates.
Haemostatic	Any substance that checks bleeding and aids the clotting of blood.
Insecticide	Any substance that is fatal to insects.
Laxative	Any substance that induces gentle, easy bowel action.
Leucorrhea	Any mucus discharge from female genitals.
Menorrhagia	Excessive flow in menstruation.
Myalgia	Any muscular rheumatic pain.
Narcotic	Any drug that induces stupor and insensibility.
Nephritic	Any drug that affects the kidneys.
Nervine	Any substance that restores the nerves to a normal tone.
Oxytocic	Any drug that contracts the uterus and hastens childbirth.

Parturient   Any product used during childbirth.

Resolvent   Any substance that reduces swelling.

Rubefacient   Any substance that produces inflammation of the skin.

Sedative   Any substance used to placate 'nerves'.

Soporific   Any substance used to promote sleep.

Stimulant   Any substance used to promote the reserve power of the body and produce strength and energy.

Stomachic   Any substance that allays stomach disorders.

Styptic   Any substance that aids the clotting of blood.

Sudorific   Any substance producing heavy perspiration.

Tonic   Any substance that, if used regularly, will promote vivacity and well being.

Vermifuge   Any substance that expels worms from the body.

Vulnerary   Any substance that promotes the healing of wounds.

FURTHER READING

Other books in this Herbal Series include:

Skin Problems
Arthritis and Rheumatism
Sexual Problems

Other Foulsham books on herbal medicine edited by David Potterton include:

Culpeper's Colour Herbal
Medicinal Plants